Boxing Footwork

Drills, Techniques, Tips & Tactics To Improve Your Boxing Power & Precision Via Footwork

1st Edition

By Frank Sasso

Table of Contents

Introduction

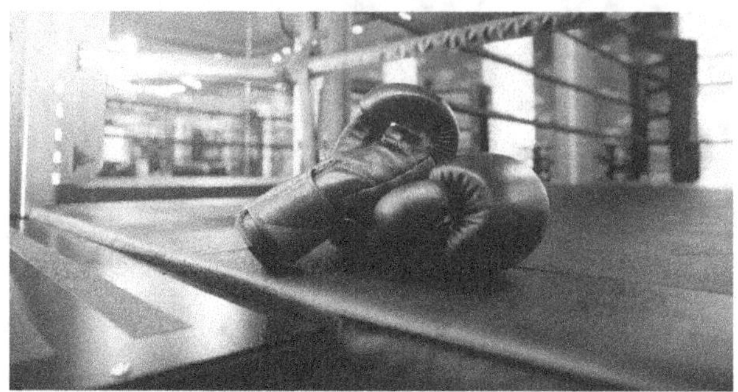

Before we delve deep into the specifics of boxing footwork I want to thank you and congratulate you for purchasing this book.

Very few people end up taking action and pursuing their goals or dreams – by obtaining a copy of my boxing footwork drills book you've taken the first step in turning your desire to improve your boxing skills into a reality.

You've spent a portion of your hard-earned cash and you've acquired what I deem to be the ultimate and only guide to improving your footwork, regardless of how limited or competent you deem your current skillset to be.

From my experience over the years the majority of guys know one or two basic boxing footwork drills, but they don't actually know how to perform them correctly or how to implement these skills in the ring...

We won't be diving straight into the boxing footwork drills though, unless you're a seasoned veteran in the ring perhaps you'd like to skip ahead to the drills which are located in chapter 6.

We'll begin by understanding exactly why developing your boxing footwork is paramount to success in the ring, then we'll shine the spotlight on some of the greats that were known to stifle their adversary's offence with their elite footwork in the ring.

After we've covered both the why and the who of boxing footwork, I'll explain how to choose the right pair of boxing boots for you (don't box in joggers! I'll explain why) before elaborating on the items you likely having laying around your house required to make these drills work.

And of course, it wouldn't be a boxing book without a primer on punches. That's right – we're going to talk about your jab, cross, hook and uppercut variations to ensure you're performing them correctly from a punching mechanics standpoint while also ensuring your striking is matching up correctly with your footwork.

Thanks again for purchasing this book, I truly hope you enjoy it!

But please remember, once you turn the last page of my book it's all on you to follow through and put the drills, exercises and techniques elaborated upon in this book to action... I can give you all the information, but YOU must put in the work...

You don't get better at any skill by not doing it.

Chapter 1 – The Importance of Footwork in Boxing

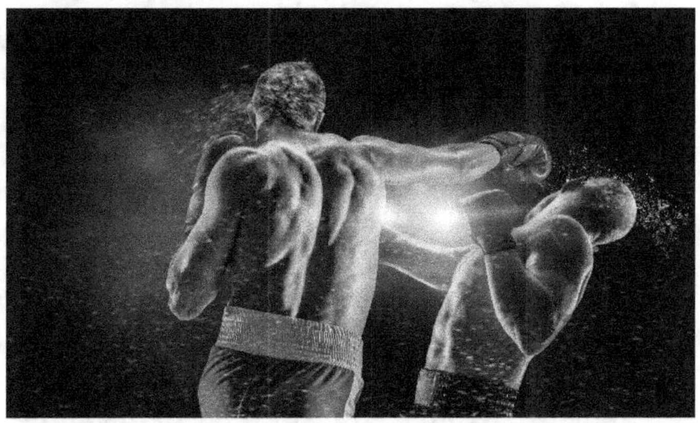

The vast majority of guys believe that boxing is all about the punching, ducking, weaving and slipping and first of all let me say I agree that footwork itself can't send your opponent crashing down against the ropes or leave them with a bad hematoma that prevents them from coming out for the next round... but it certainly sets you up to be in position to land that fight finishing combo.

Let's break down the big benefits of footwork when it comes to boxing, be it at the amateur level, professional level or even just moving around and hitting focus mitts with your friends.

Your Footwork Is The Ultimate Defense

When the topic of defense in boxing is discussed the first few thing that often comes to mind are blocks, the parry and head movement... don't get me wrong yes these are the staples when it comes to protecting yourself in the ring but at the same time with well-developed footwork you won't be in a position that'll allow your adversary to strike from an angle that would require you to block or cover up.

In later chapters of this book, I'll elaborate on some of the boxing greats with the best footwork, watch some of their fights and you'll soon see it's almost as if their opponent is fighting a ghost – one moment they're in your face teeing off with hard, well timed shots... a split second later and they're gone.

Think about it, would you rather have to cover up and weather the storm or would you rather be out of the storm's way?

Your Footwork will Allow You To Find & Exploit Angles

Great footwork creates great angles, and great angles place you in a position to land those round winning and fight finishing punches.

It's quite rare to land a knockout punch while standing directly in front of your opponent, unless you possess a sizeable speed advantage and happen to land a counter flush on your opponent's chin.

That's where angles come in. The subtle step off to the side, allowing you to blast that shovel hook to the body, the left foot pivot while you unload a check hook (pivoting lead hook) on an aggressive opponent who is attempting to back you up against the ropes.

Your Footwork Will Help You Generate Power

True power comes when you learn to sit down on your punches, in order to sit down on your punches (sinking your weight into the canvas of the boxing ring) you must be well balanced in your stance. If you're leaning forward or have your weight distribution incorrect, you'll either miss and potentially fall forward (or sideways if it's a hook that is being thrown). Sitting down on your punches and always being in a position to counter with power will come as a result of performing the drills within this book.

Think about it, if your opponent throws a wild punch and misses, leaving their chin completely exposed for a moment and you have your legs crossed over or are standing too tall you will miss your opportunity to make them pay.

Your Opponent Will Begin To Fatigue & Doubt Themselves

Trust me on this one, I've been on both sides of this statement. As a young up and comer sparring far more experienced men I would find myself with thoughts of dread, doubt and anger mid-round as I was repeatedly getting tagged by my sparring partner, every single time I tried to back them up against the corner of the ropes they'd disappear! My mind was fatigued trying to compute why I couldn't catch them and my legs were beginning to run out of gas as I hadn't put in the time performing footwork drills and roadwork like they had to build up the necessary endurance.

Now, after years of drills, road work, time in the ring and time spent studying the greats of boxing I'm the unhittable ghost. Sparring an individual that pays no attention to developing their footwork is like boxing in 3D while your opponent is only 2D. That's right, footwork adds a whole other dimension to the game.

Your opponent only sees straight lines – moving directly forward to attack and moving directly backwards to defend and retreat. You see much, much more.

Your Footwork Will Allow You To Optimize Your Energy Expenditure

Firstly, it should come as no surprise, getting hit (particularly to the body) will sap the life out of you, efficient footwork means you'll take far less damage and thus be able to optimize your energy expenditure while increasing the volume of punches being thrown per round.

Secondly, when sparring a particularly aggressive opponent (the Mexican constant forward pressure style of fighting) it can be absolutely exhausting being on your back foot for multiple rounds – instead of moving backwards in a straight line opting to use your slick footwork to cut angles will allow you to save a large amount of your gas tank while frustrating your overly aggressive adversary.

You'll Have Superior Leg Endurance From Performing Your Drills

It's all well and good that your punching and upper body endurance are on point, but in those deep dark later rounds of a bout if your leg endurance isn't up to scratch you'll find your defensive footwork becomes sloppy and you lack the energy to really sit down on your punches to do damage.

Although you may find a few of the drills repetitive and not overly fun to perform they'll be forging the leg endurance that may be the difference between you getting your hand raised and you leaving the ring with a loss on your record.

Chapter 1 Summary

- Perfect your boxing footwork and it will become your primary defense – it's far better to use your feet to escape on unconventional angles than it is to have to cover up and attempt to block, parry or weave through your opponent's punches.

- Great footwork creates angles, great angles create opportunities to land round winning and fight finishing combos.

- Learning to sit down on your punches and remaining balanced while striking both forwards and backwards will ensure you are able to place as much power behind your punches as possible.

- When your opponent can't catch you due to the evasive nation of your footwork it begins to fatigue them both physically and mentally as the rounds go on.

- Good footwork will allow you to optimize the expenditure of your energy. Fighting off the back foot is exhausting, using great footwork to pivot away and cut angles is not.

- Upper body endurance is often stressed and worked on, leg endurance is generally neglected

and can be the decider between
whether you get your hand raised
or not.

Chapter 2 – Examples of Boxers with Phenomenal Footwork

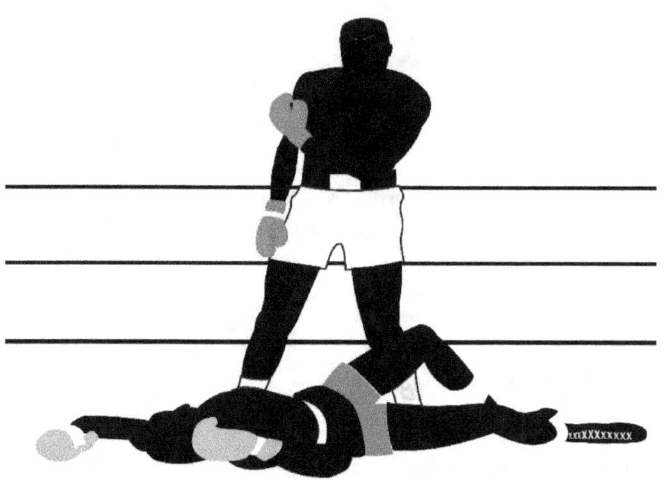

A wise boxer watches tape of his adversary before their bout to familiarize himself with his opponent's tendencies in the ring – subtle tells like dropping a hand before they throw their signature left hook, information on what they do when backed up against the rope, which direction do they like to circle? ... are they a head-hunting style of boxer? Or do they prefer to be a little bit more passive... waiting to unload that monster counter punch when you go on the offensive?

You don't have to be a competitive boxer with a bout lined up to study tape... if you truly want to take your boxing footwork to the next level, I recommend performing the drills found in the later chapters of this book while also watching displays of greatness from the following fighters. I recommend jumping onto YouTube and typing in the boxers name followed by 'highlights' or 'footwork'. Then sit back and watch poetry in motion.

You'll soon see that these top tier boxers match their footwork with their boxing style:

A head-hunting style boxer with perpetual forward motion will use their footwork to ensure they are in prime position to strike with power while ensuring they aren't in a position to end up off balance.

A defensive style boxer will use their footwork to stay slightly out of range and create angles that ensure their opponent is never able to land a clean shot or back them up into a corner of the ring.

I highly recommend checking out footage of the following boxers:

Pernell Whitaker

Take a look at any discussion on the internet regarding the boxer with the best footwork and I guarantee you'll find mention of Pernell Whitaker.

Pernell built his career on his strong defense, elusiveness and counterpunching prowess.

Pernell 'Sweet Pea' Whitaker was born on the 2nd of January 1964 and amassed a record of 40 wins, 4 losses, 1 draw and 1 no contest before passing away on July 14, 2019.

Sugar Ray Robinson

Widely regarded as the greatest boxer of all time Sugar Ray Robinson (Walker Smith Jr) was born on the 3rd of May, 1921 and amassed an outstanding boxing record of 173 wins, 19 losses, 2 draws and 2 no contests. Robinson passed away on the 12th of April in 1989.

Floyd Mayweather Jr

It's hard to argue against claims of the Floyd Mayweather Jr being the best defensive boxer to ever do it with a perfect record of 50 wins and 0 losses (27 wins coming by KO). Born February 24, 1977 at 43 years of age Mayweather continues to compete in 'exhibition' matches, with his most recent victory being over the brash Irish MMA star, Conor McGregor. Mayweather currently has a bout scheduled against Jake Paul which I cannot imagine being anything other than a one-sided beatdown.

Be sure to check out Mayweather's wins over Pacquiao and Canelo Alvarez.

<u>Muhammad Ali</u>

Cassius Clay Jr (later known as Muhammed Ali) undoubtedly the most iconic and charismatic boxer to walk this earth was known for his patented Ali Shuffle and making his opponents look like fools as they swung for the fences while Ali was nowhere to be found.

Born January 17[th,] 1942 Ali amassed a record of 56 wins and 5 losses before passing on the 3rd of June, 2016.

<u>Guillermo Rigondeaux</u>

Fast, ferocious and extremely elusive… these are all observations that'll come to mind when you watch Guillermo Rigondeaux put in work in the ring. Dubbed by legendary boxing trainer Freddie Roach as potentially the greatest talent he has ever seen. That speaks volumes.

Rigondeaux holds a professional record of 20 wins and 1 loss, that loss was to the man we're about to discuss next…

Vasyl Lomachenko

Sporting nicknames such as 'The Matrix' and 'Hi-Tech' it quickly becomes apparent that Lomachenko is not your typical head-hunting style of boxer – sporting a record of 14 impressive victories and 2 defeats Lomachenko's fastidious footwork and cutting of highly unconventional angles can without a doubt be credited to the time his father made his spend doing Ukranian dancing classes and gymnastics before his boxing career took off.

Chapter 2 Summary

- Performing boxing footwork drills is fantastic and after reading this book I highly recommend you put together a footwork regime, however just like a boxer preparing for a new opponent the importance of watching tape cannot be understated. Watch some of the technical greats in action.

- Examples of boxers to study include Pernell Whitaker, Sugar Ray Robinson, Floyd Mayweather, Muhammad Ali, Guillermo Rigondeaux, Vasyl Lomachenko

Chapter 3 – The Importance Of Boxing Boots

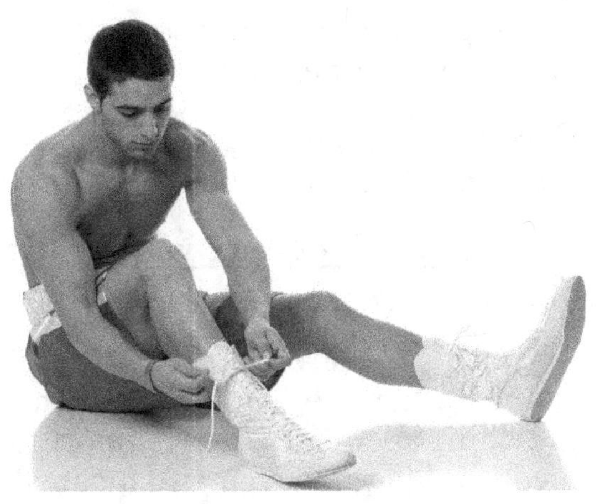

If I had a dollar for every time I've been asked about whether it's worthwhile buying a pair of boxing boots let's just say I'd probably be in the 1%… from guys jumping into one of my boxing classes for the first time to the girl that's been a workhorse in the gym for a couple of years and is now starting to take her training to the next level.

"Frank, do they actually make a difference? Is it worth dropping some hard-earned cash on pair of boxing boots?"

My answer is always the same.

It's a loud and resounding "Yes!"

Now, before we go on let it be known I don't sell boxing boots, nor do I have an affiliation with any brand that crafts them. I merely know from my own experience in the ring, from talking to others and from watching those in my classes box while wearing a pair of boxing boots that they make a huge difference.

Here's why I highly recommend you pick up a pair of boxing boots:

Boxing Boots Offer Great Ankle Support

Running shoes are made for running…they were not designed for providing adequate ankle support for fast pivots or lateral movement, meanwhile that's exactly what boxing boots were designed for. Ankle injuries can have you out of the gym and the ring for quite some time so even without considering the other benefits this is more than enough justification for me to invest my hard-earned dollars into a pair of boxing specific footwear.

Boxing Boots Make Keeping Your Balance That Much Easier When Striking

Running shoes are designed to cushion your feet with each stride, and as such you don't get a proper feel for the canvas in your boxing ring – with rigid and often chunky soles it's easy to find yourself off balance when attempting to pivot (yes,

I've fallen over in the ring trying to land a check hook while wearing my running shoes).

Purpose built boxing boots are designed with fairly thin soles that are far less rigid than most other running/training shoes – as such you have far greater feel and control of your movements making it easier to maintain your balance while sitting down on your punches, pivoting, and cutting angles.

Boxing Boots Are Designed To Fit Like A Glove

As mentioned above, the more feel you have the more control you'll have over your movements. Boxing boots are designed to be big, chunky, and decorative like many other styles of fitness/training shoes – they are thin soled, not overly rigid and are designed to fit like a glove as you don't want any unnecessary foot or ankle roll during your swift movements in the ring. You'll find most vendors of boxing shoe offer different widths and make their shoes in half sizes to ensure you can get the right size to fit like a glove.

Boxing Boots Are Literally Designed For Pivoting And Subtle Footwork Movements

From the reasonably thin and not overly rigid sole to the optimal grip pattern and precise sizing boxing boots are made to look pretty and just stand stationary...

Boxing boots are designed to be
perpetually changing direction and speed.

<u>Boxing Shoes Are As Light As A Feather</u>

Just like cycling, at the elite level every little bit of weight reduction can be the difference between first and second place. Imagine lugging around a pair of running shoes for 12 three minute rounds... regardless of how good your leg endurance is if you opt for a pair of purpose designed boxing boots (many only weight a couple of hundred grams!) you've already got yourself an advantage.

With So Many Boxing Boots Out There How Do You Choose A Pair?

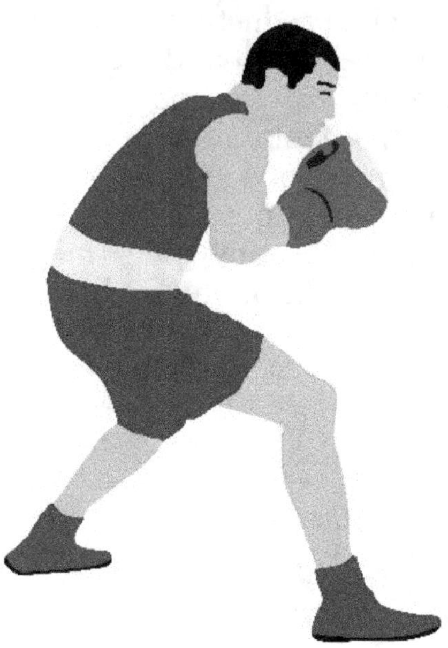

There are many brands and variations of boxing boot produced by each brand, I recommend setting a budget and trying on a few pairs of boxing boots within your budget to find what feels like the best fit for you. I personally have a narrow foot and found pivoting in a few different models of Adidas boots to be a bit uncomfortable, it didn't feel particularly natural. After speaking with some buddies at the local boxing gym I discovered that a number of the guys with a narrower foot had taken a liking to a variation of the Nike Hyper KO.

As I said, I'm not here to push a particular brand or shoe – I've personally found the shoe that fits best for me and I advise you to go out there and do the same.

You can spend anywhere from $50 for a pair of reliable Adidas boxing boots all the way up to $500 for a pair of hand-crafted Japanese Mizuno boxing boots.

Unless you're made of money or about to face off against Floyd Mayweather I believe you'll be more than satisfied with a pair of snug fitting boxing boots on the lower to mid-range of the price scale.

Chapter 3 Summary

Do boxing boots make a difference? They absolutely do. If you take your training seriously and wish to avoid injury, I highly recommend you pick up a pair – they don't need to be top of the range by any means… just find a pair that fit you like a glove.

The benefits that boxing boots offer include:

Boxing boots often fantastic ankle support during pivots, angle changes etc,

You'll feel far more grounded and maintain your balance easier while going on both the offensive and defensive in the ring.

Boxing boots are designed to fit like a glove, ensuring no unnecessary movement within your boot while cutting angles, pivoting etc.

A thin sole that isn't overly rigid with a grip pattern designed for the canvas of your boxing ring ensures you can 'feel' the canvas properly, allowing you to make minute footwork adjustments as you see fit – if you were wearing runners you wouldn't have anywhere near as much feel or control.

With most pairs of boxing boots weighing only a couple hundred grams you'll find in

long sparring sessions as you approach
the 10th, 11th and even 12th round those
light as a feather boots become a godsend
as your legs begin to fatigue.

Chapter 4 – Equipment Required for Boxing Footwork Drills

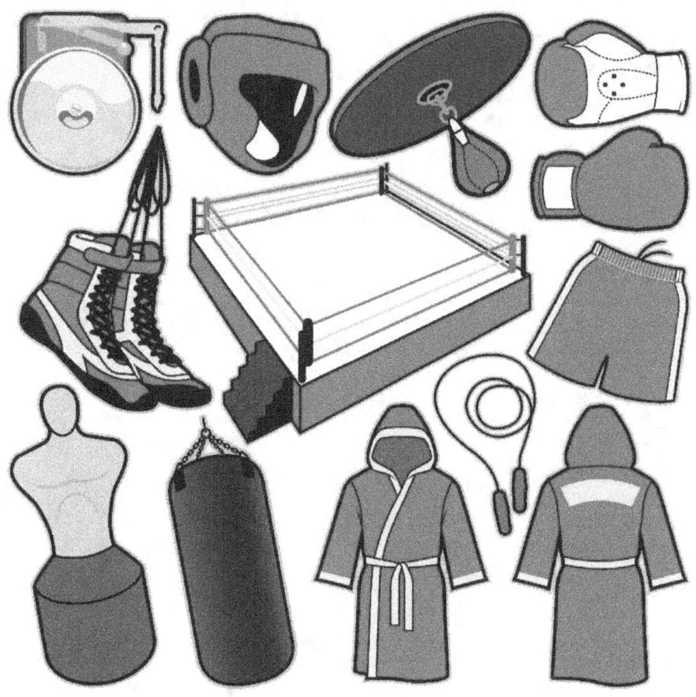

On the following page you'll find a breakdown of the necessary equipment required to perform all of our boxing footwork drills along with the purpose each individual piece of equipment will serve.

Jump Rope

The jump rope, a staple in any boxers' arsenal – not just for specific footwork drills but also for overall cardio conditioning.

When we're in the ring we want to stay light on our feet, we want to control our breathing while our heart rate begins to elevate as we move both in a straight line and laterally, we also want to remain on the balls of our feet while doing all of this – and that's exactly why the jump rope is perfect.

You can't remain flat footed or heavy while jumping rope, drills oriented around the jump rope will enforce good habits in the ring.

Cones

Half a dozen to a dozen sports cones or field markers will be used during our step in and step out drills – if you can't find field markers or sporting cones use the closest thing you can find (traffic cones are a feasible option).

We will be moving around and stepping between these cones and using the cone as a prompt to change directions, angles etc.

Tape

Ensure you are using some durable tape e.g. masking or electrical tape – preferably a different color to the flooring on which you are going to be sticking it.

We'll be using this tape as a means of position where our feet should be as we begin in our boxing stance, then where our feet should end up when we're throwing various straight punch and hook combinations.

I remember spending months day in day out in a beginner boxing class drilling these footwork drills with some tape stuck to the floor, I honestly didn't see the importance of it at the time but today looking back I'm extremely thankful that my coach put us through those tape drills – without it I wouldn't have built such a foundation of footwork early on in my boxing career.

Agility Ladder

A cheap agility ladder will do the trick – no need to buy anything fancy.
An agility ladder is a fantastic tool for building speed and lower body dexterity in any and all sports – boxing is no exception.

We'll be using our agility ladder to perform a variety of different movement patterns – going forwards, going backwards, moving laterally throughout the ladder. I personally believe the agility ladder is a great tool for training the mind too as a large amount of focus and thought are required to perform some of the more advanced drills correctly.

String

We'll be using a piece of string elevated around shoulder height to focus on pivoting, bobbing and weaving. If you've ever seen some old school boxing training footage you've likely seen a few of these string drills being performed.

Through our string drills we'll be training our footwork as well as our head movement.

Training Partner

As the late Greg Plitt said, " Champions come in pairs of two because they battle themselves in perfection." If you have access to a training partner they will without a doubt help with a number of these drills (and we'll also be incorporating some training partner specific drills). However if you're unable to find a training partner or would rather grind alone then no issues whatsoever... there will still be a ton of drills for you to perform solo.

Plyometric Box

Box jumps are one of the ultimate exercises for athletes, be it a boxer a sprinter to build the explosive leg strength required to succeed. For the sake of your shins I recommend a soft plyometric box however a ledge or similar will do if you do not have access to one of these.

Chapter 4 Summary

Some coaches out there will tell you in order to get in proper footwork training you need to spend a ton of money, and I couldn't' disagree more. In order to perform a variety of both old school and new school boxing footwork drills you will require the following:

Jump rope, cones, tape, agility ladder, string, training partner, plyometric box.

Don't have access to all of these? No worries – for example the vast majority of these drills can be performed without a training partner.

Don't have access to tape? We can use string to improvise in that particular drill and vice versa. The list above simply states ALL of the required equipment to perform ALL of the drills without making any modifications.

Chapter 5 – A Primer on Straight Punches, Hooks & Uppercuts

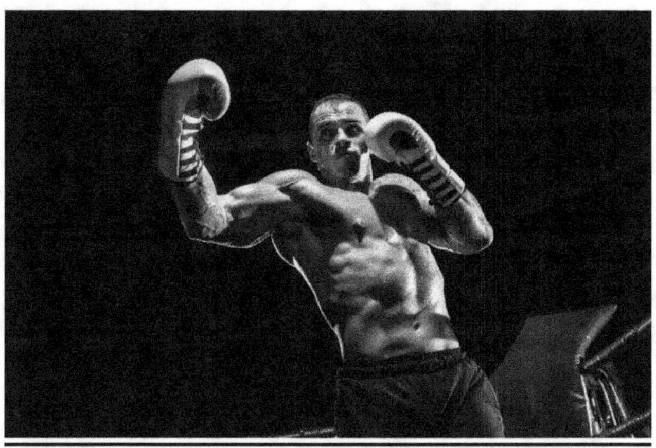

Some of the drills we'll be performing in the later chapters of this book are purely footwork, while others involve footwork while throwing strikes (on focus mitts, at a partner and while shadowboxing). As such I thought we'd go through a bit of a refresher on our punches. At the end of the day great footwork isn't anywhere near as effective if you can't make your opponent pay with well executed strikes.

Let's take a look at the jab, straight right, left hook, right hook, left uppercut, right uppercut and shovel hook.

These punches form our bread and butter, keep in mind that there are multiple variations of each of these punches (i.e. the corkscrew jab, the body jab, a tight left hook, a looping overhand right) however for the purpose of this book we'll be covering the standard variation of each of these punches.

<u>The Jab</u>

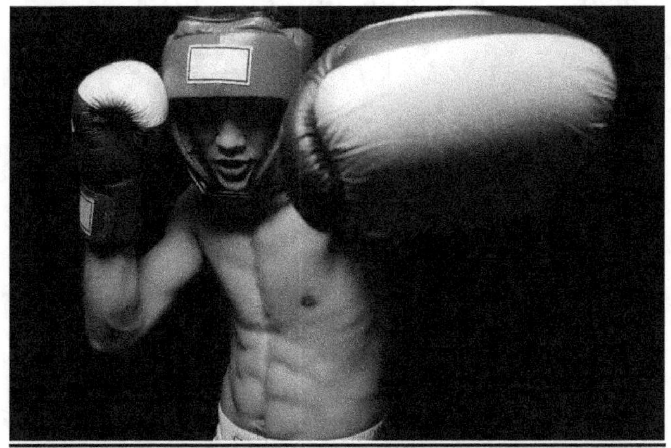

Start with your elbows tucked in (pointing down) and your gloves tucked up against your cheeks.

Extend your lead hand (left for orthodox stance, right for southpaw) as you drive through your hips.

Ensure your left hand doesn't drop at all during your punching motion – it should take the shortest path possible from in front of your face to the focus mitt/bag/opponent you are striking.

Before your arm reaches full extension rotate your fist until your knuckles are horizontal to your boxing rings canvas.

Once your jab lands bring your left glove straight back to your cheek.

If throwing a double jab instead of bringing your left glove straight back to your face opt to bring it about halfway

back before rotating through the hips once
again and throwing another jab.

The Cross

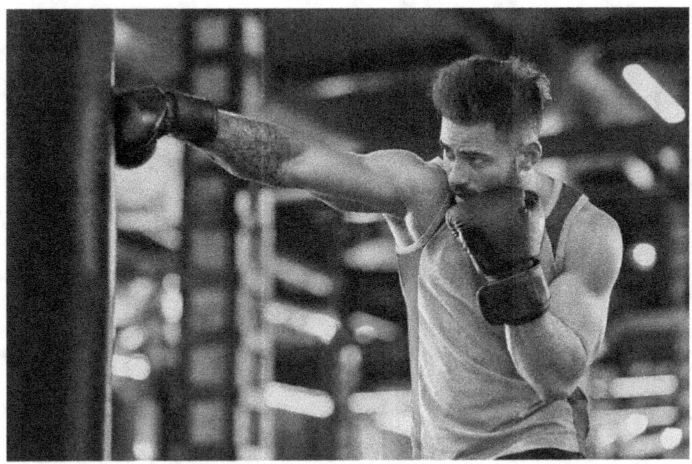

Start with your elbows tucked in (pointing down) and your gloves tucked up against your cheeks.

Extend your rear hand (right for orthodox stance, left for southpaw) as you drive through your hips.

Ensure your right hand doesn't drop at all during your punching motion – it should take the shortest path possible from in front of your face to the focus mitt/bag/opponent you are striking (this is often referred to as throwing a punch 'down the pipe').

Before your arm reaches full extension rotate your fist until your knuckles are horizontal to your boxing rings canvas.

Once your cross lands bring your right glove straight back to your cheek.

The Left Hook

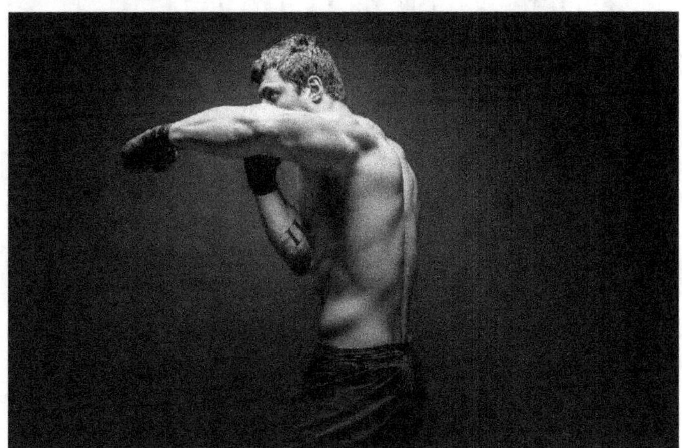

Start with your elbows tucked in (pointing down) and your gloves tucked up against your cheeks.

Begin by twisting your hips slightly to the left to load up your power.

Ensuring your left glove doesn't drop at all while doing so proceed to throw your left hand in a short hooking motion directly to your adversaries' chin, ensuring your elbow remains slightly bent. Pivot your lead (left) foot inward while twisting your hips (which should be loaded to the left) back to the right.

There's a lot of debate as to which way your knuckles should be facing when the strike lands – from my experience it comes down to personal preference... landing your left hook with your knuckles facing either horizontal or parallel to the canvas in your boxing ring is a matter of what feels more natural to you.

Once your hook lands successfully immediately return your left glove to your cheek.

<u>The Right Hook</u>

Start with your elbows tucked in (pointing down) and your gloves tucked up against your cheeks.

While pivoting on your rear right foot generate power through your hips by twisting them to the right.

Ensuring your right glove doesn't drop at all while doing so proceed to throw your right hand in a hooking motion directly to your adversaries' chin while your elbow remains slightly bent.

There's a lot of debate as to which way your knuckles should be facing when the strike lands – from my experience it comes down to personal preference… landing your right hook with your knuckles facing either horizontal or parallel to the canvas in your boxing ring is a matter of what feels more natural to you.

Once your hook lands successfully immediately return your right glove to your cheek.

The right hook is a extremely powerful and potentially fight ending punch if you're able to land it successfully, however the biggest issue is the right hook is quite easily telegraphed – your opponent can see a right hook coming from a mile away compared to your jab, straight right and left hook.

The Shovel Hook

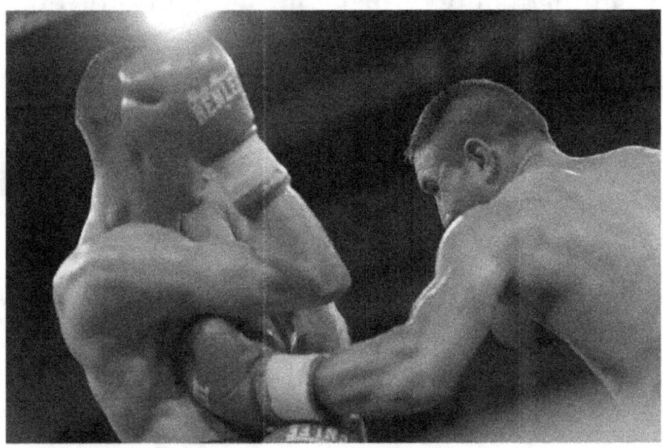

Start with your elbows tucked in (pointing down) and your gloves tucked up against your cheeks.

Take a small half step with your left foot while subtly 'loading' your hips tips to the left – this is where your devastating power is going to come from for this body shot.

Now begin to throw your left hand while pivoting back your lead foot and hips back to the right, aiming your glove for your opponent's floating rib.

There's a lot of debate as to which way your knuckles should be facing when the strike lands – from my experience it comes down to personal preference... landing your left hook with your knuckles facing either horizontal or parallel to the canvas in your boxing ring is a matter of what feels more natural to you.

Once your hook lands successfully immediately return your left glove to your cheek.

The Left Uppercut

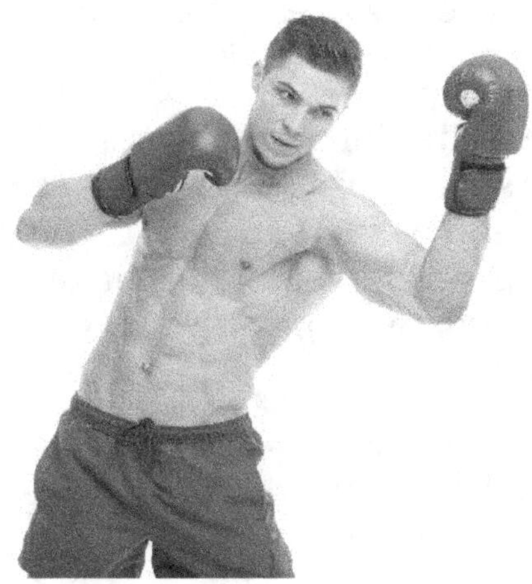

Start with your elbows tucked in (pointing down) and your gloves tucked up against your cheeks.

In one fluid motion lower your left shoulder slightly as your left glove drops down several inches (no need to lower it to your waist level) before driving through your hips and pivoting on your front (left) foot.

Fire your left glove from its slightly lowered position directly to underneath your opponents chin – generating as much power from the pivot as possible.

The second your punch lands return your left glove back to your cheek.

The Right Uppercut

Start with your elbows tucked in (pointing down) and your gloves tucked up against your cheeks.

In one fluid motion lower your right shoulder slightly as your right glove drops down several inches (no need to lower it to your waist level) before driving through your hips and pivoting on your rear (right) foot.

Fire your right glove from its slightly lowered position directly to underneath your opponent's chin – generating as much power from the pivot as possible.

The second your punch lands return your right glove back to your cheek.

Chapter 5 Summary

Summary of punches:

The Jab – a straight punch from your lead hand, often used as a range finder to land devastating power punches.

The Cross – a straight punch from your rear (power) hand. Many champions have been crowned and fortunes have been made from a powerful and accurate cross.

Hooks – The punch your opponent doesn't see coming. Statistically more knock outs have come from hook variations than any other punch. Works well as both an offensive weapon (hide a left hook behind a right cross) and as a defensive weapon (think the pivoting check hook against an aggressive opponent).

Uppercuts – When fighting in close with your opponent the uppercut is the punch of choice, with minimal space required to throw this devastating strike it works best against phone booth style fighters. A clean uppercut with power generated through the hips is enough to end even the most seasoned veterans' night if it lands flush.

Chapter 6 – Boxing Footwork Drills

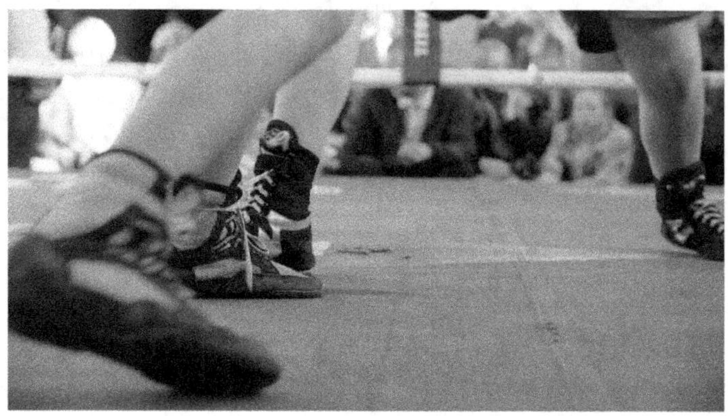

On the following pages you'll find a wide variety of boxing footwork drills that're great for beginners, intermediate boxers, and even seasoned veterans.

Regardless of whether you've spent 10 minutes or 10 years in the ring these footwork drills if performed often will take your boxing to the next level.

Boxing Footwork Drill #1 – Stance Switching Jump Rope

Begin with a jump rope, start with your left foot forward and your right foot back. With each rotation of your jump rope alternate between orthodox stance and southpaw stance (as you jump place your right foot forward and your left foot back).

Perform stance switches with your jump rope for rounds of 3 minutes.

Boxing Footwork Drill #2 – Jab Cross Forwards & Back

This was the first boxing footwork drill I was taught many moons ago and it remains a staple, as a beginner this is an excellent drill to get your punches and footwork 'connected' so to speak.

If you're a complete beginner this drill can be a little frustrating to begin with as you know what steps etc. you want to take but when you go to perform it you mis-step or throw the wrong punch.

This all comes down to repetition, spend time on this drill and you shall be rewarded.

Begin by stepping forward with your lead leg (left for orthodox, right for southpaw) while throwing a jab.

Immediately step forward with your rear leg (right for orthodox, left for southpaw) while throwing a cross.

Now that you've taken two steps forward it's time to take two steps back while repeating the same...

Step back with your rear foot (right for orthodox, left for southpaw) while throwing a jab.

Immediately proceed to step back with your lead foot (left for orthodox, right for southpaw) while throwing your straight right hand.

You should now be in the same position you started in.

Repeat for rounds of 3 minutes.

Boxing Footwork Drill #3 – The Cone 3 Punch Drill

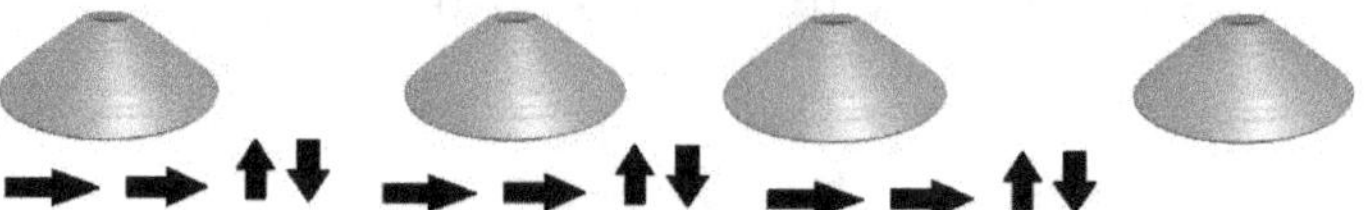

For this drill you'll need to set up 4 markers in a horizontal line with approximately 1 meter between each.

For this drill you'll be stepping in between each cone, throwing a 3 punch combo comprised of a jab, cross and left hook before taking two steps back, stepping laterally and repeating between the next cone or witches hat.

Once you've reached the end of your line of cones proceed to laterally step in the opposite direction, repeating your 3 punch combo until you're back to your starting position - this counts as 1 round.

Boxing Footwork Drill #4 – The Straight Punch Check Hook Drill

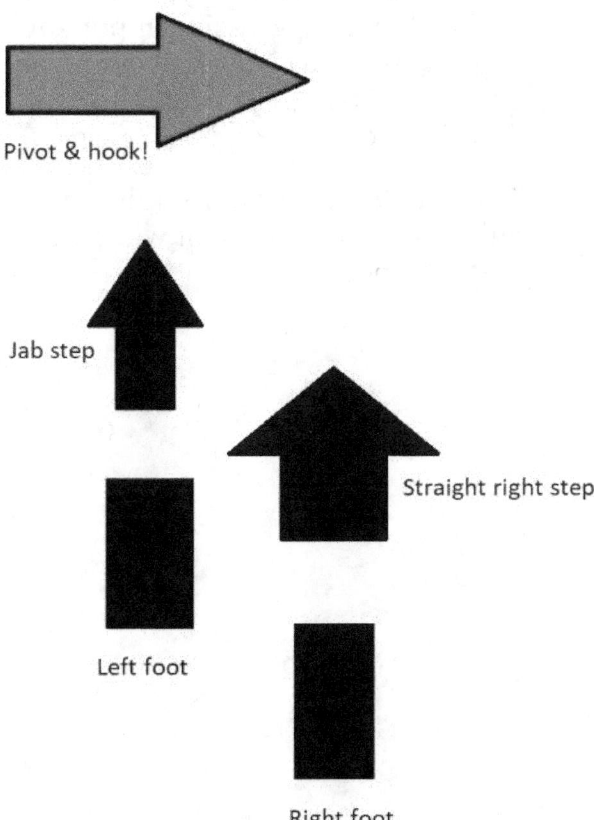

No equipment required for this drill!
Simply ensure you have a few square
meters of space to step and pivot.

Begin by taking a step forward with your
lead foot while throwing a jab, followed by

stepping your rear foot forward while throwing a straight right.

Now, here comes the fun part – the check hook.
Imagine after throwing your jab cross combo that an aggressive opponent is stepping towards you – pivot on your front foot 90 degrees while throwing a short left hook.

Continue to throw your straight punches while continuing to pivot while throwing your lead hook.

Boxing Footwork Drill #5 – Step 'N' Drag

This is a basic yet effective drill to ensure you're never caught off balance or stepping incorrectly.

Begin in your regular boxing stands with your hands up by your cheeks.

Take a step in any direction with your front on your back foot.

Swiftly slide your other foot into position so you're back in your boxing stance.

Continue to take small steps with your lead and rear foot in various direction, immediately dragging your other foot to return to your boxing stance.

However far you move with one foot is the same distance you should move with the other to ensure you're always in your optimal boxing stance.

Boxing Footwork Drill #6 – The Stance Switching Strike

I recommend performing Drill #1 with your jump rope until you are happy with your stance switching movement.

You can either perform this drill in a shadowboxing fashion or have a training partner hold a pair of focus mitts for you.

Begin in your orthodox boxing stance and take three small steps forward while throwing a triple jab – no need to place a great deal of power behind your jab in this drill, your jab should be fast and act as a range finder.

After throwing your your third jab immediately switch to a southpaw stance by stepping your right foot forward and throw a straight right (which, now you've switched stances will also be your left hand).

Regardless of whether you're a an orthodox or southpaw boxer perform this drill from both stances, switching to the alternating stance.

Either perform a stance switch from regular to southpaw and then follow up your next combo going from southpaw to regular or opt to perform 3 minute rounds of each stance switch.

Boxing Footwork Drill #7 – Plyometric Box Jumps

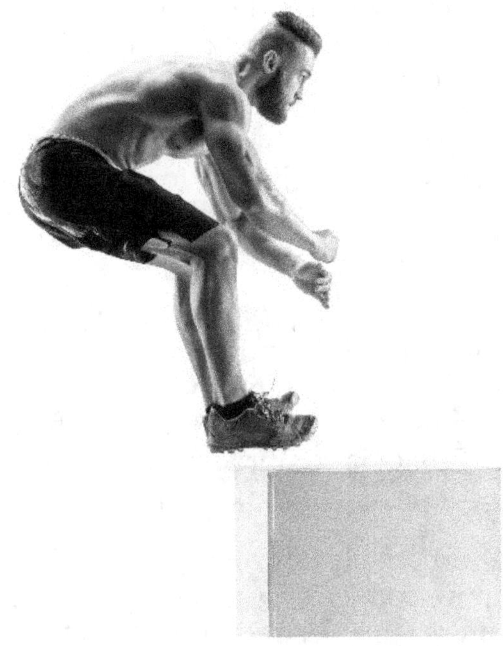

When it comes to building extreme power and speed in your legs the box jump is the go-to exercise. It's all well and good to repeat stance switching drills and the like but if your legs are lacking power and speed your adversary will take advantage of this in the ring.

I do not recommend using a metal framed plyometric box for your box jumps as I've seen far too many guys in the gym end up injured with sliced up shins thanks to these. Instead opt for a soft box that will be forgiving in case you fail to clear the box on your later repetitions as your legs begin to fatigue.

When it comes to plyometric box jumps you can perform them in various formats – for time, for a prescribed number of reps etc.

My personal favorite way to implement box jumps specifically for boxers to develop those fast explosive legs is the Tabata method.

Tabata training is a form of high-intensity interval training comprised of 20 seconds of work followed by 10 seconds of rest for a 4 minute period. Therefore, one round of Tabata is comprised of 8 rounds of 20 seconds of your box jumps.

Alternatively perform 30 seconds of box jumps followed by 30 seconds of rest until you reach a desired number of total repetitions (i.e. 100, 200).

Boxing Footwork Drill #8 – Agility Ladder In 'N' Outs

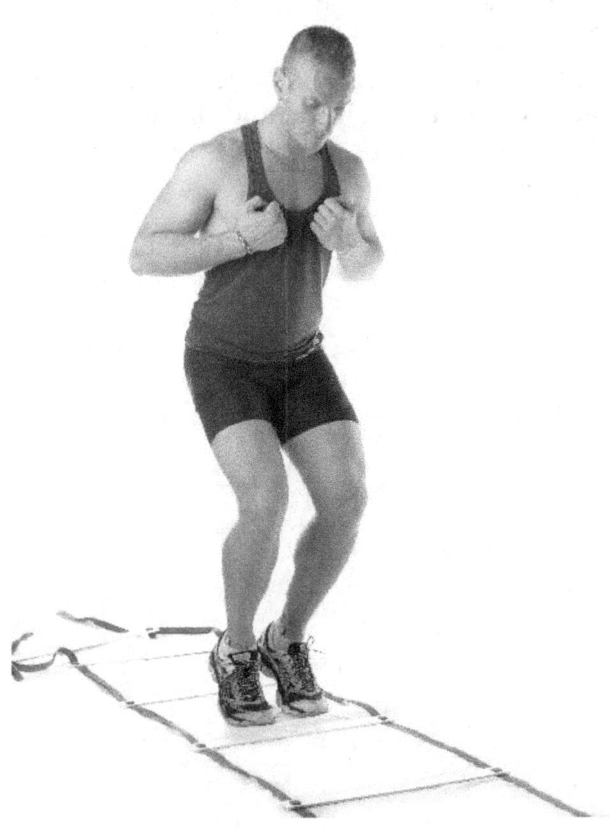

For the In 'N' Out drill you will require an agility ladder, if you don't own or have access to an agility ladder simply use some tape or chalk and draw a bunch of boxes on the floor to replicate the look of an agility ladder.

Begin with both feet inside the first square of your agility ladder before stepping outside of the ladder with your left foot, then your right foot before placing your left foot then your right foot inside the second square of your agility ladder. Proceed stepping inside and outside the squares of your agility ladder with your feet until you reach the end of the ladder, then it's time to do it in reverse (going backwards!).

Boxing Footwork Drill #9 – Agility Ladder Forward & Back

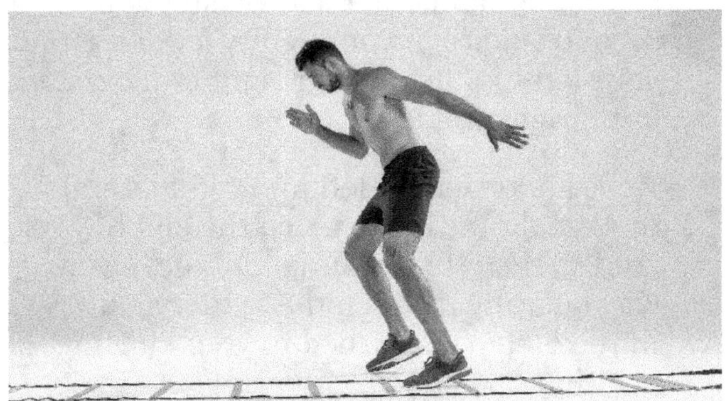

For the forward & back drill you will require an agility ladder, if you don't own or have access to an agility ladder simply use some tape or chalk and draw a bunch of boxes on the floor to replicate the look of an agility ladder.

Chances are if you've watched or participated in agility ladder drills before you've seen or performed the forward & back drill, this is a personal favorite of mine and for good reason – it's excellent for building fluidity and dexterity of movement.

Begin by standing in front of your agility ladder.

As we'll begin by moving laterally to the left side of our ladder start by placing your left foot inside the square of your ladder, as you bring your right foot into the ladder bring your left foot outside of the ladder square.

On your next step you'll be stepping first with your right foot into the second square of your agility ladder, as you step into the second square of your agility ladder with your left foot bring your right foot outside of the agility ladder.

Repeat alternating left and right lateral movement until you reach the end of your ladder, then turn around and move your way laterally through the ladder again until you have returned to your starting position.

Boxing Footwork Drill #10 – The Straight Punch Body Hook Pivot

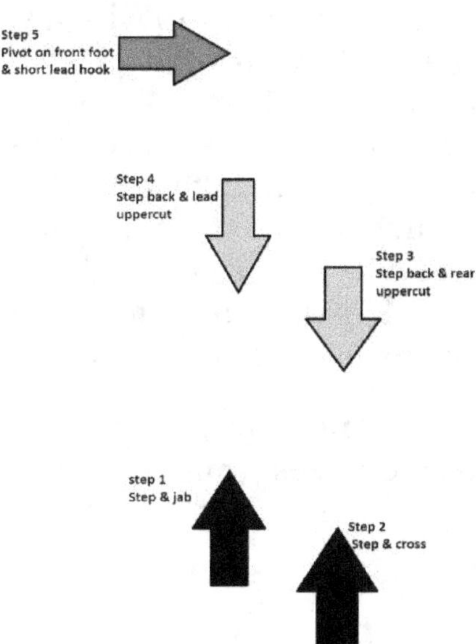

This boxing drill is comprised of a 5 punch combo that I regularly catch my opponents with in sparring, I highly recommend mastering this drill as if you're able to effortlessly punch going forwards, backwards and on a pivot you'll be trouble for any opponent in the ring… those that don't develop their footwork like you are have a pretty difficult time fighting off their back foot.

This drill can either be performed shadow boxing or on a pair of focus mitts with a training partner.

Begin in your orthodox boxing stance and take a small step forward with your left (lead) foot while throwing a jab. Immediately follow up with a small step forward with your right (rear) leg while throwing a right cross. Now we're going to pretend our adversary is on the offensive so we're going to take a step backward with our rear (right) foot while throwing a rear uppercut, then immediately taking a step back with your front foot while following up with a front uppercut.

End the combo by pivoting off to your left side 90 degrees while throwing a short left hook.

Boxing Footwork Drill #11 – The Backwards Jump Rope

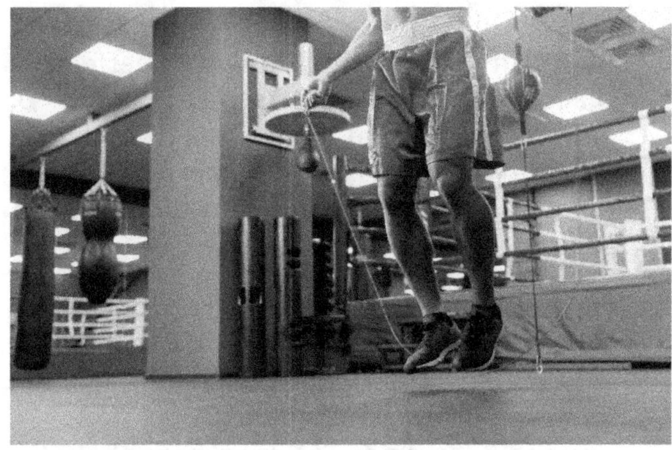

Jumping rope in the regular forward motion of the rope is easy as you can see exactly when you need to jump to clear the rope, you've got a simple visual cue... the same cannot be said for when it comes to rotating your jump rope backwards.

You have to go off of timing and feeling – both traits that must be mastered to take your boxing footwork to the next level.

I recommend performing longer rounds of 5 and 10 minutes while performing the backwards jump rope drill at a steady pace while also occasionally performing Tabata rounds of the backwards jump rope (20 seconds work, 10 seconds rest for 4 minutes).

Boxing Footwork Drill #12 – Landing The Shovel Hook

Getting hit in the face is never fun but let me assure you getting hit with a perfectly placed body shot is honestly that much worse! Speaking of body shots this drill is going to focus on landing a perfectly placed shovel hook on your opponent's rib cage.

Here's the thing – unlike our straight punches and regular left hook it's near impossible to land the shovel hook while standing directly in front of your opponent... we need to cut the right angle to blast that powerful hook to their midsection.

Here's how to do it...

Begin by throwing a jab, feinting a jab, throwing another jab and then while feinting a jab for the second time take a step to the left with your lead foot while loading your hips to the left.

From here we'll drive that lead hand shovel hook directly to where your imaginary adversaries rib cage would be.

Take a step back with your lead leg to return to your boxing stance before moving around and repeating this drill.

Boxing Footwork Drill #13 – The X

For this drill you'll require 5 cones or 5 pieces of tape placed on the floor to form a X. Essentially make a square with 4 cones and place one cone in the middle.

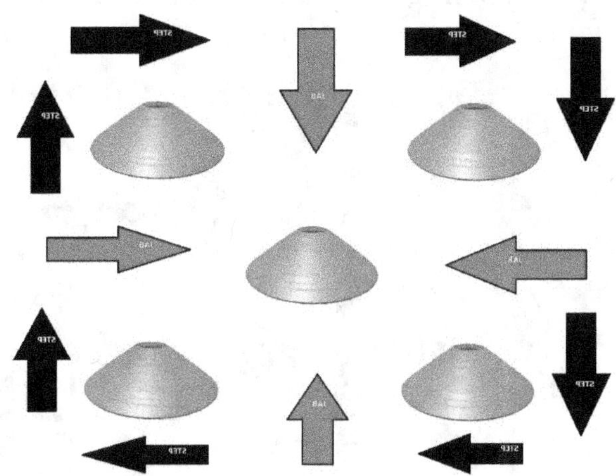

Begin by circling around your cones by stepping laterally, step in between the gap of the cones (your front foot should almost be touching the cone placed in the middle) and throw a jab before stepping back out and circling to the next opening in your cones and repeating this same jab, step out and lateral movement pattern.

When performing multiple rounds of this drill alternate the direction you are circling around the cones each round (i.e. round 1 should be clockwise, round 2 should be counter clockwise).

Boxing Footwork Drill #14 – The Cone Circle

For this drill you'll require 9 cones, witches hats or 9 pieces of tape placed on the floor. Create a circle using 8 comes while placing the 9th cone in the middle of your circle.

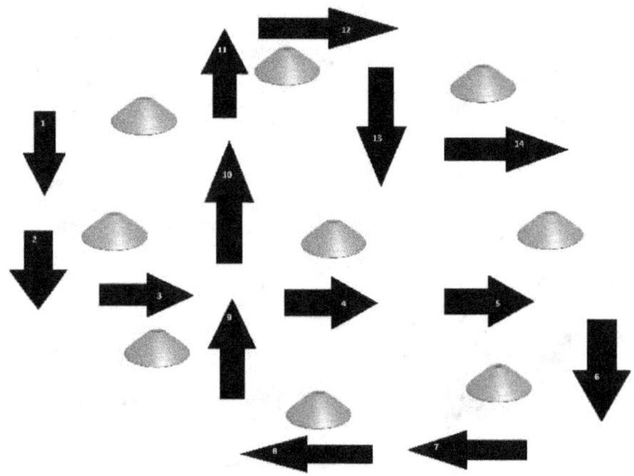

Unlike the previous 'X' drill utilizing cone which involves methodically working your way into the gap between each cone when it comes to our cone circle drill it's extremely dynamic.

That's right, we aren't going to be going in and out of each and every cone – instead opt to move laterally around the outside of some of the cones before stepping in the middle and throwing a two or three punch boxing combination of your choice before moving out the opposite side on an angle. Proceed to move around the outside of your cones again, step in and throw a combo before exiting between another set of cones on an angle and so forth.

Boxing Footwork Drill #15 – The 90 Degree Uppercut Drill

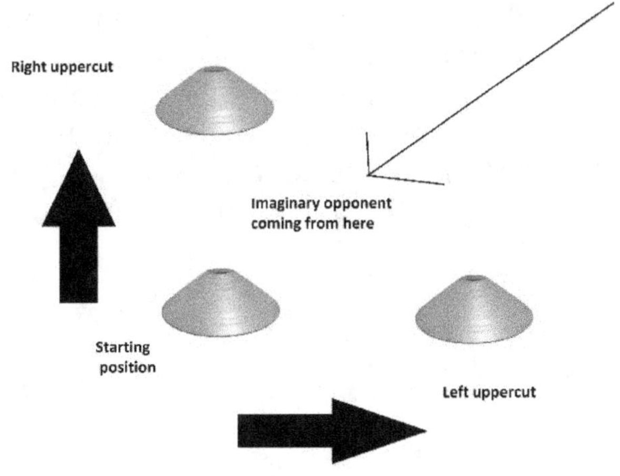

For this drill you'll require 3 cones or 3 pieces of tape placed on the floor to create a 90 degree angle (essentially the shape of the letter L).

This drill is designed to cut an angle and land an uppercut on an opponent coming towards you with straight punches – we're going to be performing this drill using both orthodox and southpaw stances.

Hop laterally from your left side of your cones to the right side of your and throw a left uppercut (the hand closest to the middle cone). Immediately hop laterally from the right side of your cones to the left side of your cones and throw a right uppercut (the hand closest to the middle cone).

Continue to repeat this drill for the desired number of repetitions, imagining your opponent is coming at you through the path of your middle cone and you're continuing to cut angles from both the orthodox and southpaw stance as you rip away with your inside uppercuts.

Boxing Footwork Drill #16 – The Tape Square Drill

For this drill you guessed it! You'll need some tape.
Begin by taping 9 squares on the floor (all joined together) each square should be approximately the size of your foot.

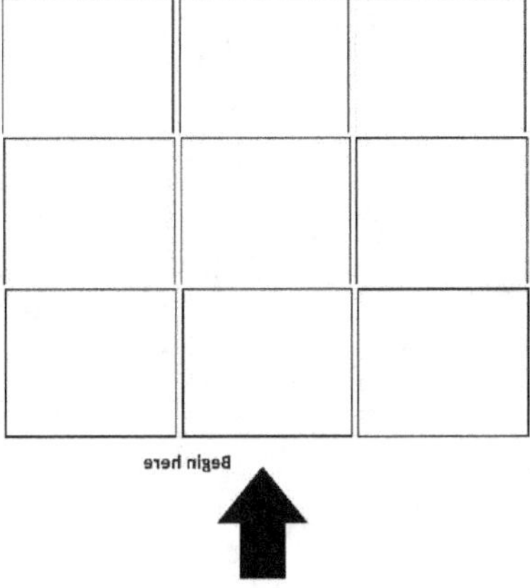

Begin standing behind the middle of the 3 squares at the back – step forward and throw a jab – your front should now be inside one of the squares. Continue to move forward, laterally to both the left and right as well as moving backwards as you step between your 9 tape squares, throwing a punch with your left hand when you step left (this could be a lead hook, left uppercut or jab) and throwing a punch with your right hand when stepping right (this could be a right hook, straight right or rear uppercut).

This is a fantastic drill to understand how far you should be stepping on each punch not to mention an excellent way to ensure you're always in your correct boxing stance after throwing a punch.

Boxing Footwork Drill #17 – The Jab Cross Puppet Drill

No equipment (or space) required whatsoever for this drill, we're going to perform this one on the spot.

The best cue to understand this drill and to ensure you're performing it correctly is to imagine that you are a string puppet. Your left hand is connected to your left foot via a string and your right hand is connected to your right foot via a string.

Begin by throwing a jab while lifting your left foot up, your left foot should return to the floor as your jab reaches its full extension. Proceed to throw a straight right hand while picking up your right foot, once again return your right foot to the floor as your straight right hand reaches its full extension.

Alternate throwing your jab and cross while lifting your left and right foot in sync with your punches.

Perform for rounds of 3 minutes.

Boxing Footwork Drill #18 – The 3 Punch Pivot

The only requirement for this boxing footwork drill is tape or some chalk to draw 4 equal sized boxes on the floor.

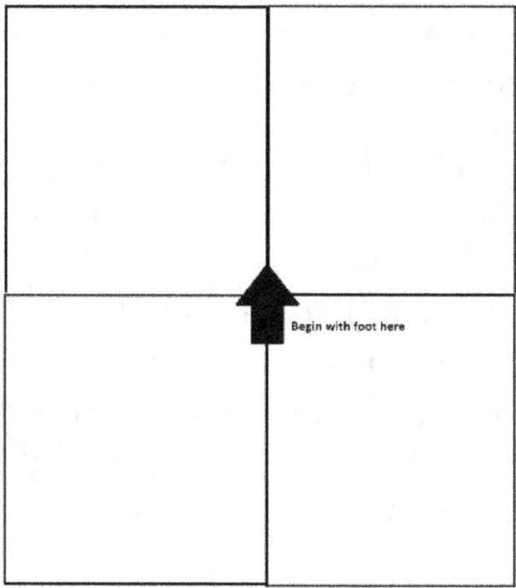

Begin in your boxing stance with your lead foot positioned on the middle line where all 4 boxes intersect. From here you'll begin by pivoting to the left on the ball of your lead foot.

Immediately throw a 3 punch combination, some examples of combos you may like to use include:

Jab – cross – left hook

Jab – jab – right uppercut

Left uppercut – right uppercut – left hook

Right uppercut – left hook – straight right

As soon as you've thrown your combo proceed to pivot again 90 degrees on your lead leg, ensuring your foot is on the middle line of the 4 boxes before throwing your next 3 punch combo.

Continue to pivot and throw a variety of 3 punch combos for rounds of 3 minutes each.

Boxing Footwork Drill #19 – Hoppers

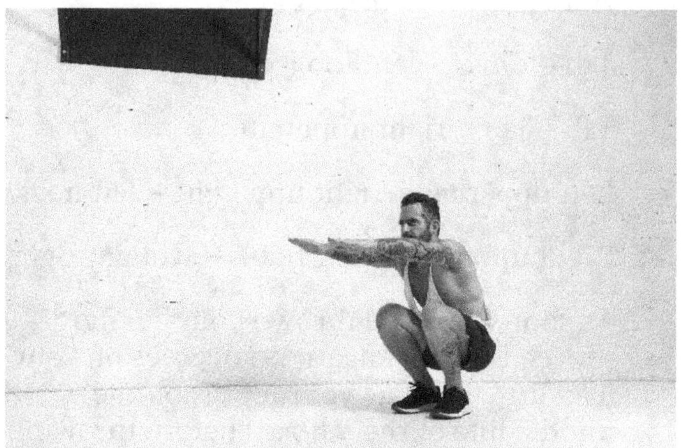

The only way to improve your endurance and current ability is to push yourself beyond your current limitations... that's what we're going to be doing with these hoppers, your quads, hamstrings, calves... your lower body is going to feel like it's on fire after a solid 3 to 5 minute set of hoppers! Push through the temporary pain and reap the rewards on the other side.

No equipment required for this footwork drill (with the exception of some mental fortitude).

Begin by dropping down low as if you were performing a bodyweight squat. Place your hands on your head and position yourself on the balls of your feet while you maintain your squat position.

Begin to perform small bounces on your toes, you can opt to remain in one spot or move around while bouncing on your toes (while remaining in your low squat position). This is one of the ultimate drills for building up that leg endurance.

Boxing Footwork Drill #20 – Shadowboxing Down Low

Once you've mastered the tough yet rewarding hoppers drill mentioned on the previous page it's time to add onto the hopping motion and add in some shadowboxing! That's right – remove your hands from your head and perform combos of between 2 and 4 punches while bouncing on your toes, opting to occasionally pivot and change directions as well as moving forward and back.

Notice how much harder it is to shadowbox down low than if you were standing?
That's the exact purpose of this drill – to put you through the hard yards in training so when you stand up and compete against an adversary your endurance, balance and movement as a whole are that much better.

Perform your shadowboxing for multiple rounds of 3 minutes while ensuring you remain bouncing on your toes in your low squat position for the duration of each round.

Boxing Footwork Drill #21 – The Ali Shuffle

Considering you're reading a book on boxing the Ali shuffle should require no introduction.
Begin with your hands held up high against your chin and begin alternating between fast and slow bursts of sliding your left foot back and your right foot forward and vice versa.

Far more than just a display of show boating, the Ali Shuffle can confuse your opponent in the ring and is a great drill to increase the speed and fluidity of your footwork.

I personally like to use the Ali shuffle in a Tabata style workout – performing 20 seconds of fast Ali shuffles before immediately performing 10 seconds of slow Ali shuffles – repeating for 4 minutes.

Boxing Footwork Drill #22 – The Slip Rope Drill

For this slip rope drill you'll need to hang a piece of string or rope that is approximately 4 metres in length at neck height, as if we set our slip rope too heigh you'll often become lazy with your head movement.

This drill is as old as the hills but is great for working on evasive footwork and head movement.

Begin on the right side of your slip rope, take a small step forward with your lead foot while throwing a jab followed by a small step forward with your rear leg while throwing a straight right.

Slip under your string or rope and take another two small steps while you throw your jab and straight right.

Proceed to slip under alternating sides of your rope while throwing your straight punches.

Once you make it to the end of the rope either opt to turn around and repeat the drill or if you're feeling up to it perform your steps, slips and straight punches while going backwards.

Chapter 7 – General Boxing Footwork Tips to Help Your Drills & Sparring

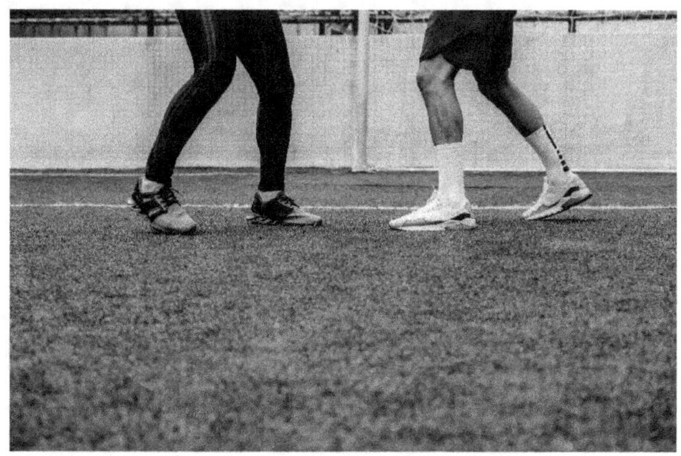

Now that you are well informed on the benefits of developing your boxing footwork, you know the advantages to wearing boxing boots, you've had a refresher on how to throw your punches correctly not to mention you've been armed with a hefty number of boxing footwork drills lets run through some general boxing footwork tips and tricks that haven't fit into any of the previous chapters.

Boxing Footwork Tip #1

Keep your body loose and relaxed.

I've coached guys with unbelievable cardio endurance when it comes to running, swimming, cycling and jumping rope... but as soon as they get in the boxing ring and start to move around with a partner they get fatigued extremely quickly.

Is this due to their cardio fitness not translating over to boxing? Not at all. It's because they're remaining extremely stiff and tense while moving around the ring.

Remaining stiff and tense is a sure-fire way to empty your gas tank in a short period of time.

Boxing Footwork Tip #2

Don't utilize too wide of a boxing stance.

It comes down to personal preference, but I personally recommend keeping your boxing stance fairly narrow – a narrow stance not only results in quicker lateral movement and pivots but it requires less energy too.

Trying to quickly change direction to get yourself off of the ropes or to pivot away from your opponent is slow, clunky and requires more energy. A lot of disadvantages and no real benefit (the only time I recommend a super wide and low stance is in the world of MMA when you have the classic striker vs. grappler match up).

Boxing Footwork Tip #3

Maintain a straight spine.

A straight spine makes maintaining your balance while striking and evading your opponent that much easier – when leaning back or hunching forward and maintaining a stance heavy on your front leg it's that much harder to remain balanced – this results in excess energy expenditure and potentially weaker punches... remember if you're off balance there's no way to sit down on your punches and really drive that power home.

Boxing Footwork Tip #4

Lower your hands when out of range (yep, you read that correctly!)

The lower your center of gravity the quicker you'll be able to move around the ring. Now, in an actual bout I do not recommend dropping your hands down if your opponent is in your face attempting to walk you down – but as you avoid strikes and move laterally around the ring you'll conserve energy and increase your footwork speed and balance by lowering them. No need to drop them down by your sides, lowering from head height to chest height will suffice.

Boxing Footwork Tip #5

Understand circling.

Using your lateral movement to circle your opponent instead of remaining a stationary target is a wise move, but you must understand which way you are circling...

Under no circumstance should you circle towards your opponent's rear hand. Circling towards their rear hand is circling into their power – allowing them to time a straight right hand (or left in the instance of facing a southpaw).

You must circle away from their power hand – I've sparred many opponents that've circled towards my power hand and I've landed devastating blows as a result (coming out southpaw then quickly switching stance and throwing power shots while your adversary is circling away from the southpaw power hand is a sneaky tactic I like to employ from time to time).

If your adversary tries to throw their rear hand while you're circling away from it they'll likely misjudge the distance and end up missing and leaving themselves wide open for a counter or missing and potentially ending up off-balance... both situations you can use to your advantage.

Boxing Footwork Tip #6

The size of the step you take with one foot is the same size you should take with the other.

This is a common mistake I see many beginner, intermediate and advanced boxers make to this day. They don't understand that in order to maintain a correct boxing stance if you step forward 5 inches with your left foot you should be stepping forward 5 inches with your rear foot and vice versa. Taking odd step sizes will result in your boxing stance being either too wide or too narrow – resulting in you missing out on an opportunity to counter your opponent or perhaps leaving you too narrow and off balance, resulting in you either being knocked down or potentially even just falling down. Not a good look.

Chapter 7 Summary

Some important boxing footwork tips and techniques to remember when performing your drills, moving around while performing focus mitt drills and while sparring include:

1 - Keep your body loose and relaxed to avoid expending unnecessary energy.

2 – Keep your boxing stance fairly narrow, allowing you to change direction swiftly.

3 – Maintain a straight spine to remain balanced while striking and evading, don't lean too far forward when on the offensive and don't lean too far back while on the defensive.

4 – Conserve your energy and increase your speed while out of range by lowering your hands from head height to chest height or slightly below.

5 – Understand circling, you must circle away from your opponent's power hand while trying to draw them onto your own.

6 – Take equal sized steps with both feet – stepping different step sizes will result in a stance that is either too narrow or too wide.

Chapter 8 – Your Boxing Footwork Workouts

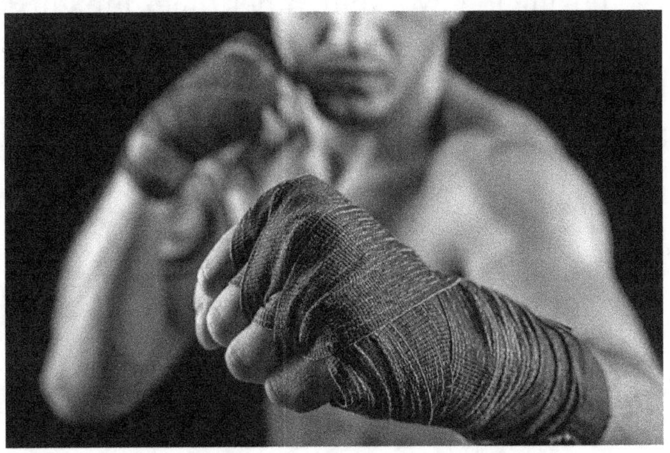

Now that I've shared with you 22 highly effective boxing footwork drills that I regularly perform and prescribe to my clients it's time to put them all together into a series of boxing footwork workouts.

Before I share my workouts with you let me start by saying these are just my examples, there's really no right or wrong way to structure your boxing footwork workout... grab a bunch of drills from this book and place them together into a workout by setting repetitions/rounds for each exercise to suit your liking.

Alternatively follow some of my examples below (sometimes I like to incorporate elements of explosive drills, endurance drills and technical drills all into one boxing foot workout, other times I might perform 3 boxing footwork workouts per week – with each workout focusing on one of these different areas.

Boxing Footwork Workout #1 – Technical Focus

Drill #3 – The Cone 3 Punch Drill – 3 rounds of 3 minutes per round

Drill #6 – The Stance Switching Strike - 3 rounds of 3 minutes per round

Drill #10 – The Straight Punch Body Hook Pivot - 3 rounds of 3 minutes per round

Drill #18 – The 3 Punch Pivot - 3 rounds of 3 minutes per round

Boxing Footwork Workout #2 – Endurance Focus

Drill #1 – Stance Switching Jump Rope – 3 rounds of 3 minutes per round

Drill #17 – The Jab Cross Puppet Drill – 3 rounds of 3 minutes per round

Drill #19 – Hoppers – 3 rounds of 3 minutes per round

Drill #20 – Shadowboxing Down Low – 3 rounds of 3 minutes per round

Boxing Footwork Workout #3 – Explosive Power Focus

Drill #7 – Plyometric Box Jumps – 5 rounds of 10 box jumps per round

Drill #21 – The Ali Shuffle – 3 rounds of 3 minutes per round

Drill #15 – The 90 Degree Uppercut Drill - 3 rounds of 3 minutes per round

Drill #8 – Agility Ladder In 'N' Outs - 3 rounds of 3 minutes per round

Drill #9 – Agility Ladder Forward & Back - 3 rounds of 3 minutes per round

Boxing Footwork Workout #4 – Well Rounded

Drill #10 – The Straight Punch Body Hook Pivot - 3 rounds of 3 minutes per round

Drill #5 – Step 'N' Drag - 3 rounds of 3 minutes per round

Drill #3 – The Cone 3 Punch Drill - 3 rounds of 3 minutes per round

Drill #7 – Plyometric Box Jumps – 5 rounds of 10 box jumps

Drill #8 – Agility Ladder In 'N' Outs - 3 rounds of 3 minutes per round

Boxing Footwork Workout #5 – Well Rounded

Drill #2 – Jab Cross Forwards & Back - 3 rounds of 3 minutes per round

Drill #11 – The Backwards Jump Rope - 3 rounds of 3 minutes per round

Drill #13 – The X – 3 rounds of 3 minutes per round

Drill #22 – The Slip Rope Drill – 3 rounds of 3 minutes per round

Conclusion

Thank you again for purchasing my boxing footwork drills book!

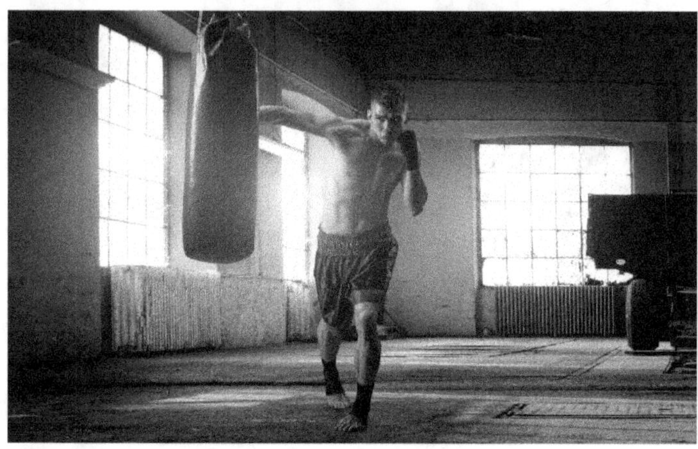

I hope you've found this book to be valuable; I can still vividly remember the day I stepped foot in a boxing gym with a dusty old pair of Everlast gloves that I picked up from a yard sale down the road from my parents' house.

As I mentioned in the introduction of this book I can equip you with all the knowledge in the world on how to improve your boxing footwork but it's up to you to put this newly acquired knowledge to work with the techniques, tactics and drills you've now become familiar with.

Lastly, if you enjoyed this book I'd be ever
so grateful if you could share your
thoughts in a review on Amazon.com. It'd
be greatly appreciated.

Best of luck on your journey my friend,
now go out there and start grinding.

Frank Sasso.

Want To Build An Unbreakable Mindset?

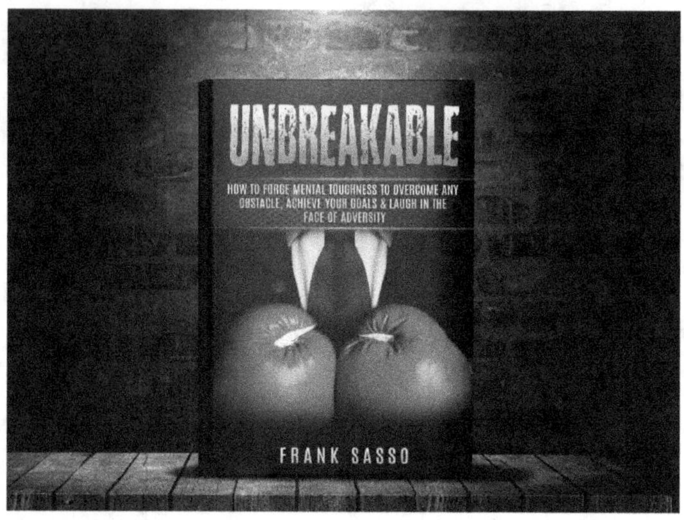

Available now on Amazon in both Kindle & paperback variants.

https://www.amazon.com/dp/B08S2Z4Q88

How About Killer Grip Strength?

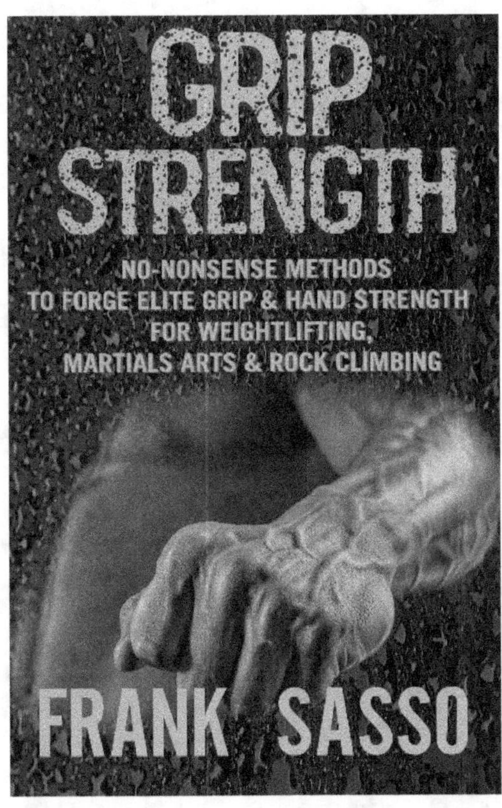

Available now on Amazon in both Kindle & paperback variants.

https://www.amazon.com/dp/B08SQDK6J9